Built From the Inside

How Smart Food Choices Create Stronger, Faster Athletes

Ray Stone

Email: **info@raystonebooks.com**
Phone: **(470) 563-5055**
Web: **www.raystonebooks.com**
IG/X: **RayStonebooks**

© Copyright 2025
Raymond Stone LLC
All Rights Reserved
Without prejudice UCC 1-308 (old 1-207) & 1-103

No part of this book may be reproduced without formal, written permission – per contract with two human signatures.

Manufactured in the US Republic (Northwest Amexem)
10 9 8 7 6 5 4 3 2 1
For Library of Congress Data, See Publisher

Pregame Meal

Built From the Inside
You are what you eat.

Disclaimer

This book is for educational and informational purposes only.

The information shared in Built Different is not intended to replace professional medical advice, diagnosis, or treatment. Always consult with a qualified healthcare provider, athletic trainer, or medical professional before making changes to diet, training, recovery, or physical activity—especially if you have an existing medical condition or injury.

The author is not responsible for any injuries, losses, or damages that may result from the use or misuse of the information in this book. Readers assume full responsibility for their actions and decisions.

Use common sense. Listen to your body. When in doubt, seek professional guidance.

Introduction

Most athletes focus on what you can see.

    Muscles.
    Speed.
    Highlights.
    Stats.

Very few think about what's happening on the inside.

    What you eat.
    How your body recovers.
    How clear your mind feels.
    How long your body can hold up.

That's where the real difference is made.

Being Different Isn't Easy

Let's be honest.

Eating differently than your friends isn't easy.
Saying no when everyone else says yes isn't easy.
Choosing discipline when shortcuts are everywhere isn't easy.

You might get jokes.
You might get questioned.
You might feel like you're doing too much.

That's normal.

Most people choose what's easy in the moment.

Athletes who last don't.

Discipline Is a Skill

Discipline isn't something you're born with.

It's something you practice.

Every time you choose:

- Better food
- Better hydration
- Better recovery

You're training discipline.

That skill doesn't end when the game ends.

It follows you into:

- School
- College
- Careers
- Life

What you build now stays with you.

Coaches and Recruiters Notice More Than Talent

Talent gets attention.

Habits get trust.

College coaches and recruiters look for athletes who:

- Take care of their bodies
- Stay consistent
- Handle pressure
- Make smart decisions

An athlete who fuels and recovers properly stands out.

Not because they talk about it.
Because they live it.

This Book Is About Advantage

This is not a diet book.

It's not about perfection.
It's not about extremes.
It's not about labels.

It's about learning how food choices affect:

- Energy
- Recovery
- Focus
- Performance

It's about gaining an edge where most people aren't paying attention.

While others are eating whatever is easiest, you're building something stronger from the inside.

Built From the Inside Wins in the End

Being different can feel uncomfortable now.

That discomfort is training.

The habits you build today create the athlete you become tomorrow.

> Strong bodies last longer.
> Clear minds perform better.
> Disciplined athletes separate themselves.

This book is for athletes who are ready to take responsibility for what goes into their bodies — and what comes out of their effort.

Welcome to **Built From the Inside**.

Built From the Inside Menu

Snack #1........12
The Edge Starts Before the Game

Snack #2........24
Learning the Lesson Early

Meal #1........36
Food Changes How Your Body Feels

Meal #2........44
Recovery is Part of Performance

Snack #3........52
What You Drink Matters More Than You Think

Meal #3........60
Simple Food. Real Control.

Meal #4........70
Playing the Long Game

Final Plate........86

Snack #1
The Edge Starts Before the Game

Most athletes think preparation starts when the game starts.

Or maybe when warmups begin.

Real preparation starts earlier.

It starts with what you put into your body.

Everyone Wants the Same Results

Everyone wants:

- More energy
- Faster recovery
- Better performance
- Fewer injuries

But most athletes follow the same habits.

They eat what's easiest.
They drink what's popular.
They recover when something hurts.

That's why most athletes get the same results.

The Edge Is in the Details

The biggest advantages in sports are rarely obvious.

They're quiet.

They show up in:

- How your body feels late in games
- How fast you recover between practices
- How clear your mind stays under pressure

Food plays a role in all of that.

Not as a rulebook.
Not as perfection.

As information.

Food Is Information

Everything you eat sends a message to your body.

Some foods say:
  Recover faster.
  Stay light.
  Stay clear.

Other foods say:
  Slow down.
  Hold inflammation.
  Crash later.

Your body listens either way.

Most Athletes Learn This Late

Many professional athletes admit the same thing.

>They didn't care about food early on.
>They could get away with it.

Until they couldn't.

>Injuries lingered.
>Recovery slowed.
>Energy dipped.

That's when food became serious.

You don't have to wait that long.

Being Different Is a Choice

Eating differently than your teammates isn't easy.

It can feel awkward.
It can feel isolating.
It can feel unnecessary.

At first.

Discipline always feels uncomfortable before it feels normal.

Discipline Builds Identity

Every disciplined choice does more than help your body.

It builds:

- Focus
- Confidence
- Self-control

Those traits don't disappear when the game ends.

They follow you.

Coaches and Recruiters Pay Attention

Talent gets noticed.

Consistency gets trusted.

Athletes who take care of their bodies stand out.

   Not because they talk about it.
   Because they show it.

   Discipline shows up in posture.
   In energy.
   In availability.

That matters.

This Book Is About Advantage

This isn't about being perfect.

It's about being intentional.

It's about learning how food choices affect:

- Performance
- Recovery
- Longevity

It's about building strength from the inside.

✍️ Write It Down

When do you usually eat without thinking?

What foods make you feel light and energized?

What foods make you feel heavy or sluggish?

Where could one small change give you an edge?

_____

_____

_____

_____

23

Snack #2
The Shortcut Most Athletes Miss

Most athletes don't start out disciplined.

They start out talented.

Talent carries them for a while.

Early Talent Can Hide Bad Habits

When you're young, your body is forgiving.

You can:
- Eat anything
- Sleep late
- Skip recovery

And still perform.

For a while.

That's why many athletes don't change early.

They don't feel the cost yet.

Maturity Changes the Game

As athletes get older, something shifts.

> The body doesn't bounce back the same way.
> Recovery takes longer.
> Small injuries stick around.

That's when habits start to matter.

Athletes don't change because they want to.

They change because they have to.

The Best Athletes Get Smarter, Not Just Stronger

Great athletes don't just train harder as they age.

They train smarter.

> They clean up their food.
> They pay attention to recovery.
> They listen to their bodies.

Not because it's trendy.

Because it works.

Starting Early Is a Quiet Advantage

Here's the shortcut.

You don't have to wait for:

- Injuries
- Burnout
- Setbacks

You can start now.

When you build smart habits early:

- Your body lasts longer
- Your energy stays consistent
- Your recovery improves

You separate without working more.

Discipline Feels Different When You're Young

When you're young, discipline can feel unnecessary.

Why change if things are working?

Because what works now won't always work later.

The athletes who last don't wait for problems.

They prepare for them.

Getting Older Isn't the Goal – Getting Wiser Is

Athletes don't improve just because they age.

They improve because they learn.

You don't need more years.

You need better habits.

This Is How You Skip Steps

Most athletes go through this same cycle:

- Talent
- Overuse
- Injury
- Adjustment

Smart athletes shorten the cycle.

They are smart enough to adjust early.

That's the shortcut.

What You See Isn't Always What They Do

You might see your favorite athletes in commercials.

Fast food.
Sugary drinks.
Bright packaging.

It looks normal.

But here's what most people don't talk about.

Those athletes are hired to advertise.

That doesn't mean they eat that food.

There's a Difference Between Promotion and Preparation

At the highest levels, teams have:

- Chefs
- Nutrition staff
- Recovery specialists

Many top athletes also work with personal nutritionists.

They understand what helps their bodies perform.

Advertising is part of business.

Fueling the body is part of the job.

Those are not the same thing.

Don't Copy the Commercial – Copy the Habits

It's easy to copy what you see on TV.

It's harder to copy what happens behind the scenes.

What actually separates athletes is:

- What they eat consistently
- How they recover
- How they prepare

Not what they promote.

Learn the Lesson Early

Most athletes don't learn this until later.

You don't have to wait.

You can enjoy sports culture without copying every habit that comes with it.

Smart athletes know the difference.

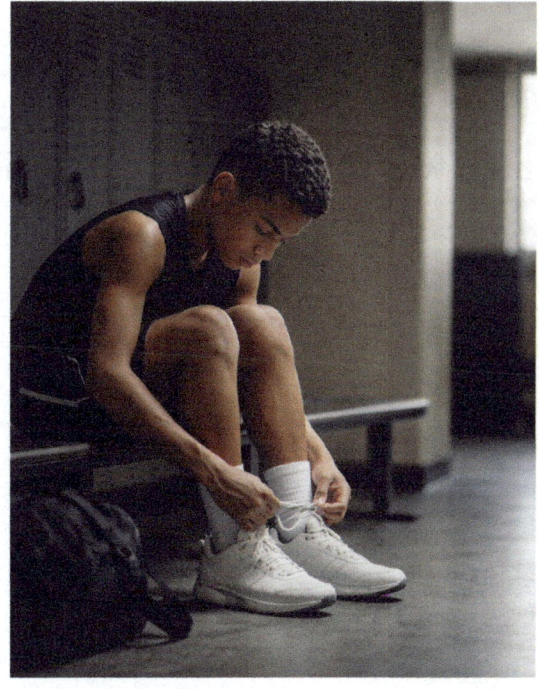

✍️ Write It Down

What habits do you rely on just because you're young?

What do you think older athletes wish they changed sooner?

What is one habit you can start now that will help you later?

What habits do you see publicly that might not match what happens behind the scenes?

_____

_____

_____

Meal #1
Food Changes How Your Body Feels

Food isn't just fuel.

It's feedback.

Every meal tells your body something.

Heavy Fuel vs Light Fuel

Some foods feel heavy.

You eat them and feel:

- Slower
- Tired
- Stiff
- Foggy

Other foods feel lighter.

You eat them and feel:

- Clear
- Loose
- Energized
- Ready

That difference matters in sports.

Why Heavy Food Holds You Back

Heavy foods take longer to break down.

They sit in your body.

Energy gets pulled toward digestion instead of performance.

You might not notice it right away.

But late in games, it shows up.

Light Food Works With Your Body

Light foods digest faster.

They give your body what it needs without weighing it down.

Athletes who feel light:

- Move more freely
- Recover faster
- Stay sharper longer

This isn't about eating less.

It's about eating smarter.

Pay Attention to How You Feel

You don't need a rulebook.

Your body already gives you feedback.

After you eat, ask yourself:

- Do I feel energized or sluggish?
- Do I feel loose or tight?
- Do I feel clear or foggy?

Patterns show up quickly when you pay attention.

Be aware of your patterns and use that data as an advantage.

The Game-Day Guideline

Before practices and games, choose food that feels light.

That doesn't mean perfect.

It means intentional.

Heavier foods can wait.

Simple, Low-Stress Choices

You don't need complicated meals.

Simple foods often work best:

- Easy-to-digest meals
- Foods that don't slow you down
- Foods that leave you feeling ready

Athletes who feel good move better.

Most Athletes Learn This Later

Many athletes don't think about food until:

- Energy drops
- Recovery slows
- Injuries linger

You don't have to wait.

Awareness is the shortcut.

One Change Is Enough

You don't need to change everything.

One better choice before activity.

One adjustment at a time.

That's how habits stick.

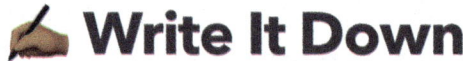 Write It Down

What foods leave you feeling heavy?

What foods help you feel clear and ready?

What is one small change you can try before your next practice or game?

_____

Meal #2
Recovery Is Part of Performance

Most athletes think recovery starts when something hurts.

That's too late.

Recovery is part of the work.

Training Breaks the Body Down

Every practice and game creates stress.

> Muscles tear slightly.
> Joints take impact.
> The nervous system gets taxed.

That's normal.

Growth happens during recovery.

Why Soreness Lingers

Sometimes soreness fades quickly.

Other times it sticks around.

That usually means the body hasn't fully recovered.

Not because you're weak.

Because recovery didn't get enough attention.

Inflammation Is a Signal

Inflammation isn't always bad.

It's part of healing.

But too much inflammation slows things down.

It shows up as:
- Stiffness
- Swelling
- Lingering aches
- Tight movement

How you treat your body affects how fast inflammation settles.

Food and Recovery Are Connected

What you eat after activity matters.

Some foods support recovery.

Others make the body work harder.

This isn't about blame.
It's about understanding cause and effect.

Recovery Isn't Just Rest

Recovery includes:

- Sleep
- Stretching
- Hydration
- Light movement
- Post-game care

Ignoring recovery doesn't make you tougher.

It shortens careers.

Professionals Don't Skip This

At higher levels, recovery is non-negotiable.

Athletes stretch before and after games.

They ice sore joints.

They take care of small issues early.

Not because they're fragile.

Because they want to stay available.

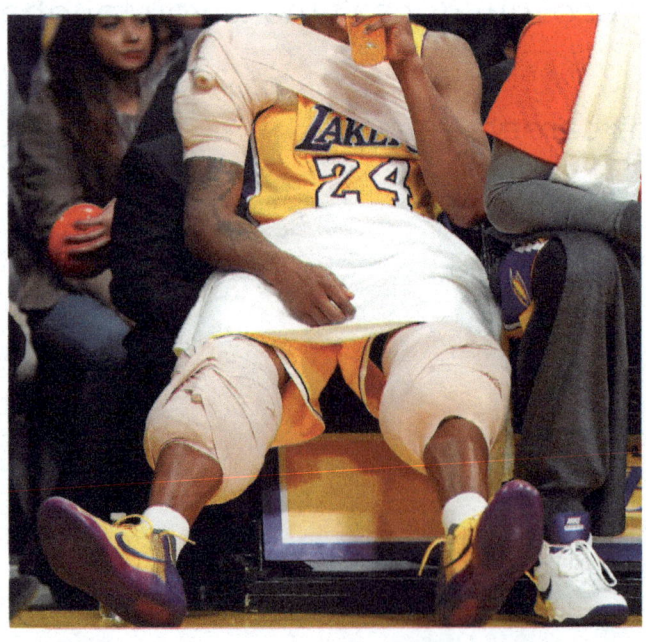

Availability Is a Skill

The best ability is availability.

Athletes who can practice consistently:

- Improve faster
- Earn trust
- Stay in rotation

Recovery helps you stay on the field or court.

You Don't Have to Do Everything

You don't need expensive tools.

Simple habits make a difference:

- Stretching regularly

- Cooling down properly
- Sleeping enough
- Paying attention to soreness

Consistency beats intensity.

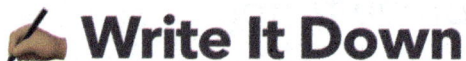 Write It Down

Where do you feel soreness most often?

What do you usually do after games or practices?

What is one recovery habit you could improve?

_____

_____

Snack #3
What You Drink Matters More Than You Think

Most athletes think about food.
Very few think about what they drink.

That's a big mistake.

Hydration Is Performance

Your body is mostly water.

When you're dehydrated:
- Energy drops
- Focus slips
- Muscles tighten
- Recovery slows

Even small dehydration affects performance.

Thirst Comes Too Late

By the time you feel thirsty, your body is already behind.

Hydration isn't something you fix during the game.
It's something you build way before it starts.

Salty, dry snacks like chips or fries pull water out of the body and make it harder to stay hydrated without realizing it.

Carrying water with you makes hydration automatic.

I keep a water bottle with me daily because it helps me drink more without thinking about it.

Not All Drinks Help

Some drinks hydrate.

Others look like they do.

Bright colors and sweet flavors don't equal performance.

Many popular sports drinks are designed to:

- Taste good
- Sell well

Not necessarily to help your body recover or perform better.

Simple Works Best

Your body doesn't need complicated formulas.

It needs:

- Water
- Minerals
- Balance

Athletes have hydrated successfully long before modern packaging existed.

A Smarter Game-Day Drink

Some athletes and families make simple drinks at home.

A basic option might include:
- Water
- Citrus

- A small amount of natural sweetness
- A pinch of salt

Nothing fancy.

Just something that replaces what you lose when you sweat.

Pay Attention to How You Feel

After drinking something, notice:

- Do you feel refreshed or sluggish?
- Does your stomach feel calm or heavy?
- Do you feel steady or jittery?

Your body gives feedback here too.

Hydration Helps Recovery

Drinking well doesn't just help during the game.

It helps after.

Hydration supports:

- Muscle recovery
- Joint comfort
- Energy the next day

Skipping hydration makes everything harder.

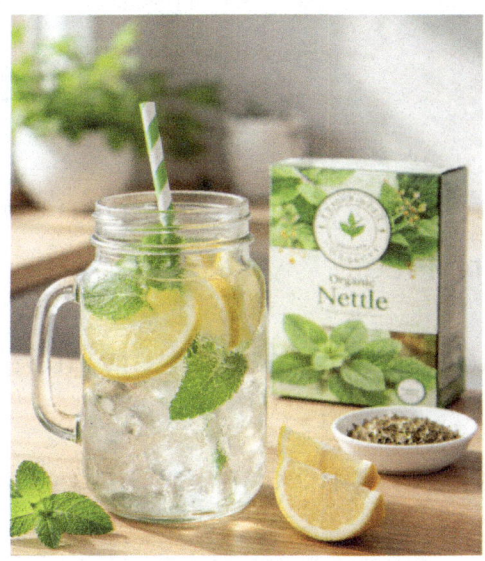

Make It a Habit

You don't need to overhaul everything.

Start by:

- Drinking water consistently
- Paying attention to how drinks affect you
- Choosing simple options more often

Small habits make a big difference.

✍🏽 Write It Down

What do you usually drink during games or practices?

How do you feel afterward?

What is one change you could make to hydrate better?

Meal #3
Simple Foods. Real Control.

You don't need permission to take care of your body.

You don't need a chef.
You don't need fancy meals.
You don't need to know how to cook.

You just need awareness.

Taking Responsibility Starts Small

At some point, every serious athlete learns this:

What you eat is your responsibility.

Not your coach's.
Not your parents'.
Not your teammates'.

Yours.

You are in control.

The sooner you learn that the better.

Simple Food Still Works

You don't need complicated meals to eat better.

Simple foods often work best.

Foods that:

- Digest easily
- Don't slow you down

- Help your body recover

This isn't about being perfect.

It's about being intentional.

No Cooking Required

There are foods you can prepare yourself right now.

No stove.
No recipes.
No experience.

Examples include:

- Salads made with lettuce, tomatoes, and cucumbers
- Fruit bowls

- Oatmeal
- Smoothies

That's real food.

And it's enough to make a difference.

Simple Add-Ins That Matter

Some athletes add small things to their meals to support recovery and energy.

Whole foods like:

- Hemp hearts
- Chia seeds
- Flax seeds
- Oats
- Frozen fruit

These are:

- Easy to find
- Easy to use
- Safe for all ages

They add nutrition without making food heavier.

Where These Fit

You can add them to:

- Smoothies
- Oatmeal
- Yogurt
- Salads

You don't need everything.

One or two additions done consistently is enough.

This Is Where Discipline Shows

Choosing simple food isn't always popular.

   It might look boring.
   It might feel different.
   It might get comments.

That's part of discipline.
Discipline doesn't always look exciting.
It looks consistent

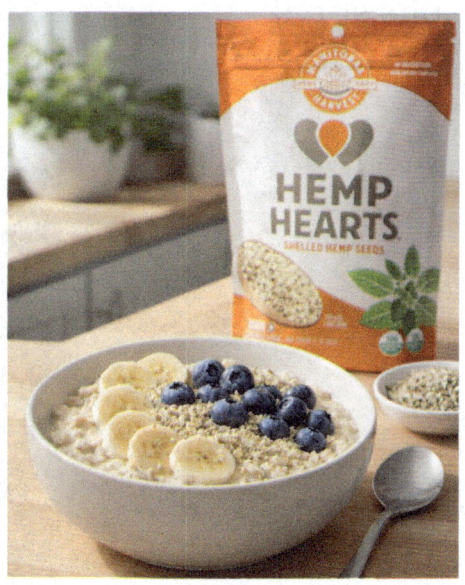

Food Choices Are Quiet Leadership

When you take care of your body:

- People notice your energy
- They notice your availability
- They notice your consistency

You don't have to explain anything.

Results speak.

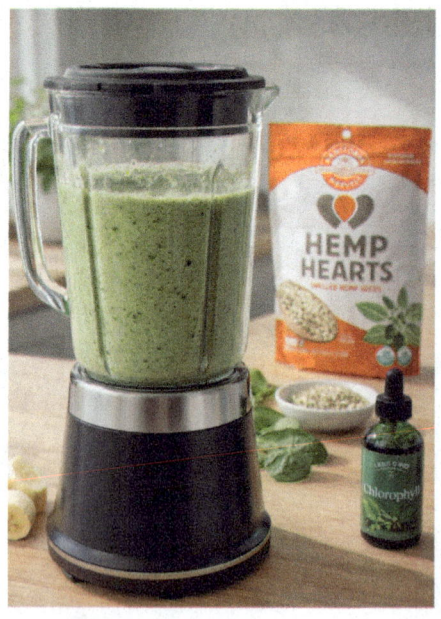

This Is an Edge You Can Control

You can't control:

- Playing time
- Team politics
- Other people's effort

You can control:

- What you eat
- How you hydrate
- How you recover

That control adds up.

✍️ Write It Down

What foods can you prepare yourself right now?

What simple add-ins could you start using?

What food choice would help you feel lighter and more prepared?

_____

_____

_____

_____

Meal #4
Playing the Long Game

Everyone loves the highlight.

Very few people talk about what happens after.

Talent Gets You Noticed. Habits Keep You Playing.

Talent opens doors.

Habits decide how long they stay open.

Athletes who last don't rely on talent alone.

They take care of their bodies.

Your Athletic Prime Is Shorter Than You Think

Every athlete has a window.

It opens.
It peaks.
It closes.

How you treat your body affects how long that window stays open.

Small choices made early matter more than big changes made late.

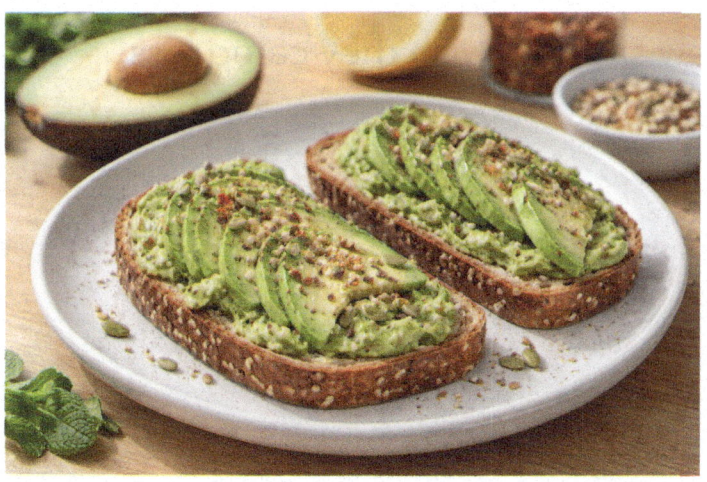

Most Regrets Come From What Was Ignored

Ask older athletes what they wish they did differently.

You'll hear the same things:

- Took recovery more seriously
- Paid attention to food earlier
- Didn't push through everything
- Listened to their body

Very few say they wish they cared less.

Being Different Early Pays Off Later

It's not easy to stand out when you're young.

Doing things differently can feel uncomfortable.

But comfort doesn't build careers.

Discipline does.

The habits you build now separate you later.

Longevity Is a Skill

Playing longer isn't luck.

It's preparation.

Athletes who last:

- Recover well
- Eat intentionally
- Stay consistent

They don't wait for problems.

They plan for them.

This Applies Beyond Sports

Discipline doesn't disappear when sports end.

It follows you.

The same habits that:

- Protect your body
- Sharpen your focus
- Build consistency

Help you succeed in life.

You Don't Need to Be Extreme

You don't need to be perfect.

You don't need to change everything.

You just need to care earlier than most people do.

That alone puts you ahead.

The Quiet Advantage

Most athletes chase what's visible.

The real edge is quiet.

It shows up in:

- Energy
- Availability

- Focus
- Longevity

Those who understand this early don't have to explain themselves.

Their careers do it for them.

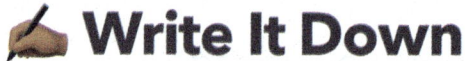 Write It Down

What kind of athlete do you want to be remembered as?

What habits will help you last longer?

What is one choice you can make today that your future self will thank you for?

_____

Built From the Inside

By now, you understand something many athletes don't.

Performance isn't just about effort.

It's about preparation.

This Was Never About Perfection

You don't have to eat perfectly.

You don't have to do everything right.

You just have to be more aware than most.

Awareness changes outcomes.

Small Choices Create Big Results

What you eat.
What you drink.
How you recover.

Choosing brightly colored drinks less often and making something simple instead.

These choices don't seem big in the moment. But they are a step.

Over time, they add up.

That's how separation happens.

Discipline Is a Form of Respect

Taking care of your body is a form of respect.

Respect for:

- Your talent
- Your time
- Your future

Athletes who respect their bodies last longer.

Being Different Is Part of the Path

You may not always blend in.
You may make choices others don't understand.

That's okay.
Leadership often means going first.

This Is a Skill You'll Always Have

Sports don't last forever.

Habits do.

The discipline you build now will help you:

- In college
- In careers
- In life

That's a win no matter what level you play.

You Don't Need Approval

You don't need to explain your choices.

You don't need to convince anyone.

   Your energy.
   Your consistency.
   Your availability.

Those will speak for you.

Built From the Inside Wins

Strong bodies last longer.

Clear minds perform better.

Disciplined athletes separate themselves.

What you build on the inside shows up on the outside.

Every time.

✍️ Final Write It Down

What is one habit from this book you will keep?

What does "built from the inside" mean to you?

What kind of athlete (and person) are you becoming?

_____

_____

_____

_____

Final Plate

You don't need to rush this.

Progress happens one choice at a time.

>Stay curious.
>Stay disciplined.
>Stay aware.

Your body is your Temple.

Strive to put good things inside.

That's how you build from the inside.

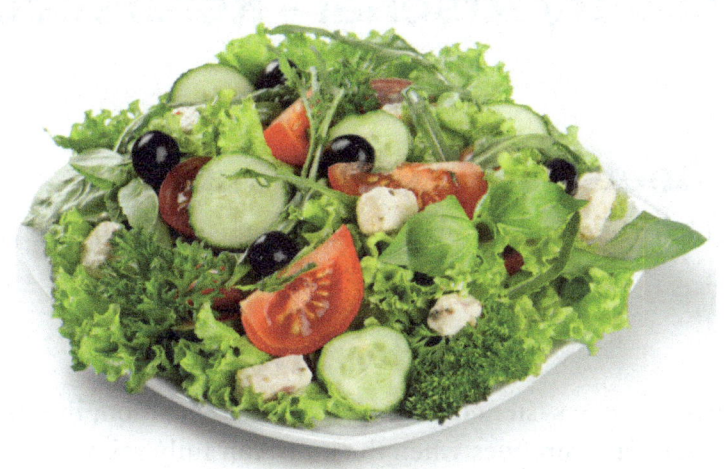

Simple fuels well.

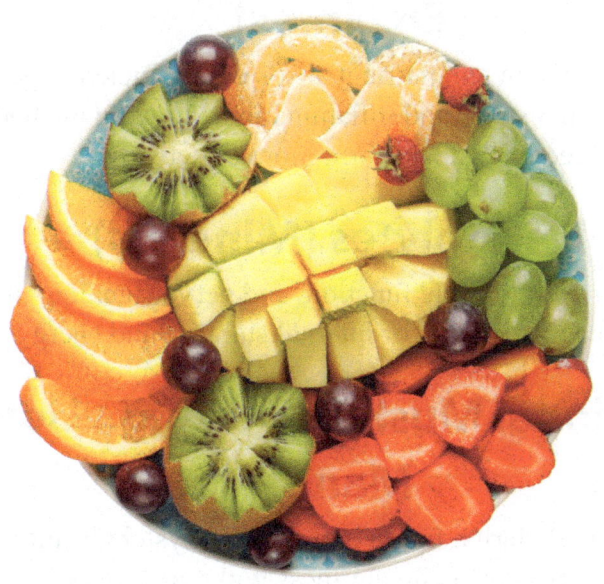

Recovery Arsenal – Reference Guide

Beets (Nitric Oxide Support)

Support blood flow and circulation, helping the body move oxygen and nutrients more efficiently.

Breathwork

Supports nervous system balance and stress regulation; internal recovery improves when the body can fully relax.

Digestive Support (Probiotics / Enzymes)

Supports digestion and nutrient absorption; efficient digestion reduces internal stress and inflammation, allowing the body to recover and perform more effectively.

Electrolytes (Minerals)

Support hydration, muscle function, and nerve signaling; mineral balance is essential for internal stability and energy.

Functional Mushrooms (e.g., Lion's Mane)

Support mental clarity, focus, and nervous system health; often used to promote calm alertness without stimulation.

Folate (Vitamin B9)

Supports red blood cell production and oxygen delivery; important for circulation and cardiovascular efficiency.

Magnesium

Supports muscle relaxation, nervous system balance, and sleep quality; often used to help the body fully unwind.

Sleep

Primary window for physical and internal recovery; the body repairs, balances hormones, and restores energy during deep rest.

Tart Cherry

Supports recovery and sleep; may help reduce internal inflammation and soreness following intense activity.

Too Much Stimulation

Constant stimulation from coffee, energy drinks, or pre-workouts can keep the body tense; digestion, sleep, and recovery work better when the body can slow down.

Turmeric (Curcumin)

Supports joint health and internal inflammation balance; commonly used to aid recovery without reliance on NSAIDs.

Many of these tools are explored in greater depth in later works focused on nutrition, recovery, and longevity.

The Thinking Athletes Series

Built From the Inside is part of a growing collection of books designed to help athletes think more clearly about their bodies, preparation, and long-term success.

Each title explores a different aspect of athletic development, from recovery and discipline to food and longevity, helping athletes build careers that last.

About the Author

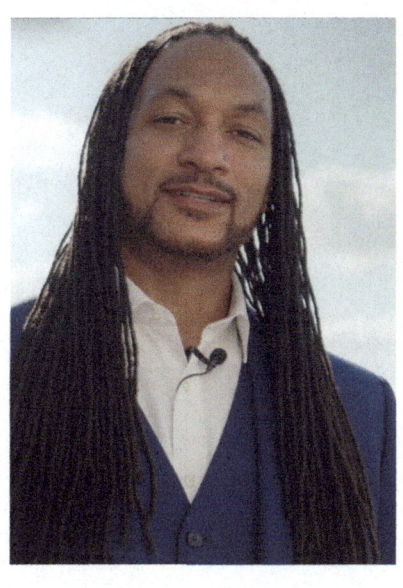

I'm Ray Stone, an author and former hooper from Detroit, Michigan. Basketball gave me opportunities, but my attitude and lack of discipline limited how far my career could go. I didn't understand early on how short an athletic prime really is, or how important it is to take care of your body like a professional. **Built From the Inside** is the guide I never had. One that helps athletes understand their body, protect their energy, and build habits that support performance and longevity from the inside out.

Made in the USA
Coppell, TX
11 February 2026